Diets to help
GLUTEN AND WHEAT ALLERGY

Rita Greer, herself experienced in coping with gluten and wheat allergy, recognizes the problems faced by the exclusion dieter. Here is sound practical advice on foods to avoid and also useful sections containing menus and recipes for gluten- and wheat-allergic patients.

This book is intended as a background to the subject, for general interest and to introduce aspects of the special care required in following this kind of diet.

GW00598462

Also in this series:

Diets to help
GLUTEN
AND WHEAT
ALLERGY

RITA GREER

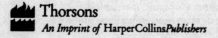
Thorsons
An Imprint of HarperCollinsPublishers

Thorsons
An Imprint of HarperCollins*Publishers*
77–85 Fulham Palace Road,
Hammersmith, London W6 8JB
1160 Battery Street,
San Francisco, California 94111–1213

First published as *Diets to Help Coeliacs
and Wheat Sensitivity* 1982
This edition, revised and updated, 1993
10 9 8 7 6

A catalogue record for this book
is available from the British Library

ISBN 0 7225 2910 4

Phototypeset by Harper Phototypesetters Limited,
Northampton, England
Printed and bound in Great Britain by
Caledonian International Book Manufacturing Ltd, Glasgow

Contents

Introduction

GLUTEN AND WHEAT ALLERGY – AN UNSOLVED MYSTERY

In the West, we have used wheat and, to a lesser extent, rye, barley and oats as a basic part of our daily diet for thousands of years. It seems odd, therefore, that some of us are unable to cope with such food and that by eating it some people can be made really ill.

Why this should be so remains a mystery. Fortunately for these people, by avoiding consumption of wheat, rye, barley and oats, good health may be enjoyed again. On paper it seems to be a very simple remedy. In real life, which is geared to the ordinary person, quite able to keep healthy while eating those four grains, the situation is more difficult. Fitting a special diet into family life can cause problems, both on the kitchen front and with shopping.

THE DIFFICULTIES OF SPECIAL DIETS

A special diet can be regarded as a 'fad' by many people. Eating out may be so fraught with problems that it has to be largely avoided and this may also be taken to be anti-social behaviour. Very often the diet must be followed for life and cannot be considered in the same way as, say, a weight-reducing diet where breaking the rules merely postpones the effect of the diet. Eating wheat, rye, barley or oats when they should be avoided can lead to adverse reactions and a return to illness.

WHO THIS BOOK IS FOR

Some patients are only adversely affected by a part of the wheat, rye, barley and oats, i.e. the gluten that these grains contain. Others may be affected by the whole of one or more of the grains.

For practical purposes, this book excludes the whole of the four grains. The two main related illnesses which can benefit from this type of exclusion diet are coeliac disease (gluten sensitive) and wheat sensitivity (or allergy). Dermatitis herpetiformis patients are also known to benefit from such dietary measures.

HOW THIS BOOK CAN HELP

This book attempts to answer the kind of questions which the exclusion dieter usually asks when faced with a complete turnabout in eating habits, and to provide practical help and advice in the form of:

- lists of 'safe' and 'unsafe' foods
- suggested menus (including some emergency ones)
- recipes

The author has been involved in a ten-year research programme on gluten-free and wheat-free foods and has also written five gluten-free and wheat-free cookery books. In addition, she has formulated many specialized foods for UK manufacturers and, through cooking regularly for just such a gluten- and wheat-free dieter, has gained valuable practical insight into the problems such people face.

WARNING

In this book, certain brand names of foods are mentioned. This is because, within a whole range of items readily available, such as soy sauces, there are some which contain gluten/wheat (usually the majority) and some which do not. However, manufacturers can change their formulas at any time and it is a sensible policy to check the ingredient list of every food that you buy just to make sure there has been no change. Brand names are only included in this book as a helpful guide where difficulties may arise with shopping.

NOTE FOR WHEAT-FREE DIETERS ONLY

Although wheat-free dieters may be able to tolerate rye, barley and oats, these are rarely found on their own in commercial products; e.g. rye bread usually contains a good proportion of wheat, as do some rye crispbreads. It is essential to *check ingredient labels* on foods. One product which wheat-free dieters will find useful and very easy to obtain is rye crispbreads. However, if this is too heavily relied upon, the diet can become boring, and crispbread is not a substitute for bread made with yeast.

NOTE FOR THOSE FOLLOWING A GLUTEN-FREE AND LACTOSE-FREE DIET

Some people who are allergic to gluten are also allergic to *lactose* (found in milk). All the special flours in this book are lactose-free and can be used safely.

CHAPTER ONE

Some Facts on Coeliac Disease, Gluten and Wheat Sensitivity

Since coeliac disease and gluten/wheat sensitivity are quite different it is as well to look at a few facts about them in simple terms.

Coeliac disease is known by a variety of names such as: non-tropical sprue, idiopathic steatorrhoea, gluten enteropathy. (In the USA, coeliac is spelt 'celiac'.) It is pronounced 'see-lee-ack'. It is not an infectious disease. Diagnosis is usually based on 'clinical features' and a jejunal biopsy. This may be superseded by a much easier test in the next few years. The disease often shows up in infants at the weaning stage but it can be diagnosed at any age.

COELIAC DISEASE

History

Attention was first drawn to this disease as long ago as 1888. The cause remained a mystery and the disease was known as Chronic Intestinal Infection (C.I.I.).

Curiously, children with C.I.I. in Nazi-occupied Holland *improved* when all Dutch wheat was sent to Germany. When this stopped, the health of the children *deteriorated* again. It was 1950 before gluten (in the wheat) was finally proved to be the culprit. The condition was by this time named coeliac disease.

Gluten

Gluten is part of the elastic, rubbery protein found in wheat, barley, oats and rye. It is the part of the grain which binds the dough in baking. Flours that do not contain gluten do not behave in the same way and a binder has to be added in order that it may be used for baking. As well as being used for

- bread
- cakes
- biscuits
- pastry

gluten-rich flour is used widely in the food manufacturing industry as a thickener and cheap filler. Therefore, gluten can be present in items such as

- gravies
- soups
- sauces
- pickles

- instant puddings
- sweets
- chocolates

Gluten is *added* to some flours, particularly for bread making, to make them 'strong'.

Consequences for Health

Much of what we eat, including fat and vitamins, is absorbed through the surface of the small intestine via the villi. These are tiny fronds which line the organ and help to give an absorption area of about ten square metres in an adult. The villi themselves are covered with microvilli (called the brush border) which increase the total area to about 300 square metres and make the small intestine even more efficient.

In coeliac disease, the small intestine becomes so damaged by gluten that the villi become flat and cannot do their job of absorbing nutrients. Not surprisingly, an untreated coeliac fails to thrive and becomes mal-

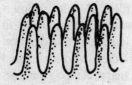

normal villi (fronds)

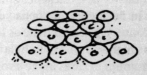

damaged villi as in coeliac disease

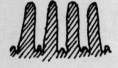

section through villi

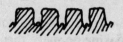

section through damaged villi

nourished. After weaning, coeliac children fail to grow satisfactorily and are thin and wasted looking. Patients are weak and listless.

Treatment

For coeliacs there is no drug treatment or cure. Fortunately, if gluten is removed from the diet, the small intestine may return to normal function, in time. In some patients, gluten must be avoided for life, but in others this need not be so.

Incidence

The incidence of coeliac disease varies from country to country. It is said to be as low as 1 in 6500 in Sweden and as high as 1 in 230 in Ireland. In children, about an equal number of cases in the two sexes is usual. Among patients diagnosed in later life, there are about twice as many women as men sufferers.

GLUTEN AND/OR WHEAT SENSITIVITY

Symptoms

People can be allergic or sensitive to gluten and/or wheat and have quite a different set of symptoms from the coeliac patient. Physical symptoms can include:

- slight to severe muscle stiffness
- aches
- redness and swelling of the joints
- sneezing
- eye-watering
- stuffy and runny nose
- chest pains
- nausea
- stomach pains and cramps
- swollen stomach
- bloated feeling
- sweating
- tiredness
- skin rashes and itches
- throat troubles
- swallowing difficulties
- swollen throat

Psychological symptoms are:

- apathy
- irritability
- depression
- moodiness
- confusion

Other symptoms may involve:

- blackouts
- flushing
- anxiety
- nervousness
- chilling
- 'the jitters'
- asthma

Diagnosis

Diagnosis is usually by blood or skin test, firstly with abstinence from gluten/wheat and then with a 'challenge'. Sometimes just a rotated diet is used in conjunction with close monitoring of the severity or disappearance of symptoms. Wheat is high on the list of foods which may cause allergic reactions. It has been shown as one of the most likely causes in triggering migraine attacks in clinical trials in the UK.

Treatment

Some research has been carried out on the use of desensitizing drops and drugs which can mask allergy symptoms for a short period. However, most experts agree that if a person is allergic or sensitive to gluten/wheat, the best course of action is to stop eating gluten/wheat.

Sometimes people 'recover' from wheat allergy and can begin to take gluten/wheat again. Children can 'grow out of it' too. Many people need to leave it out of their diet for life.

CHAPTER TWO

Questions Answered

Most people, faced for the first time with a gluten-free/wheat-free diet, either panic or become desperate for help. Many find difficulty in obtaining the information they need. They try all kinds of sources; the local library, the nearest hospital, the local health shop, bookshops, a medical charity. They are bound to experience difficulty over what is a problem that affects only a small minority of the population. Inability to obtain the necessary information can lead to frustration and distress as the days go by.

Once the health problem has been recognized and the patient realizes that many changes in former eating habits are necessary, the answers to the following questions need to be understood and some may have to be memorized. If the patient is only a young child, then the parents or guardians will need to take responsibility for changes in his diet. The child should be taught gradually, as he or she grows older and becomes capable of understanding the problem, how to cope.

Q. What is gluten?

A. Gluten is part of the *protein* found only in some grains.

Q. Which grains contain gluten?

A. The four gluten-containing grains are:
- wheat
- rye
- barley
- oats

Q. What does gluten do?

A. Gluten acts as a rubbery kind of binder when liquid is added. Without gluten, baking would just produce heaps of crumbs.

Q. Is gluten necessary for health?

A. No. Everyone could live a perfectly healthy life without ever eating gluten.

Q. What are wheat, rye, barley and oats used for?

A. They are used for home and commercial baking; breads, cakes, biscuits, pastries, buns, breakfast cereals, etc. It does not matter if the colour of the flour is brown or white – they all contain gluten. If you see a flour labelled 'strong', this means extra gluten has been added to make it bind more. The gluten-containing flours are also used as fillers and extenders, to make foods go further and to bind mixtures, by manufacturers of puddings, pastes, spreads, sweets, pills, etc.

Q. What does going on a gluten- and wheat-free diet entail?

A. It means not eating any product which is likely to contain gluten from wheat, rye, barley and oats. This means that many home- and commercially-baked products must be avoided as well as certain items from the grocer, supermarket, sweet shop, fish shop and butcher.

Q. Which basic foods are gluten- and wheat-free?

A. • Butter, cooking oils and margarines that do not contain wheat-germ oil
- Eggs (fresh)
- Milk and plain cheeses such as Cheddar and Cheshire
- Fresh fish (plain)
- All fresh vegetables
- All fresh fruit
- All fresh nuts
- Fresh meat (plain)
- Rice (plain)
- Wine or cider vinegar
- Sugar

Q. How can I do baking?

A. You must avoid wheat and rye flours, barley and oat meals. You must use naturally gluten-free and wheat-free flours instead.

Q. Which flours are naturally gluten-free and wheat-free?

A. Soya flour, maize flour, yellow split pea flour, rice flour or ground rice, tapioca, arrowroot, sago flour, potato flour and Trufree brand flours. These are all naturally gluten- and wheat-free.

Q. Do these naturally gluten-free flours bind like ordinary flour?

A. Trufree flours bind well as they have a binder added. The rest bind very poorly, but can be used with binders such as dried pectin, grated apple, methylcellulose and egg white.

Q. Can I get by without doing any special baking?

A. Yes, but you may find the diet a bit lacking in variety as your main sources of starch will be limited to potatoes, rice and bananas. You may lose weight as, unless careful, you could take insufficient carbohydrate and protein in your new diet.

Q. Are there other items I will have to be careful about?

A. Pepper

Although the purchase of *pure* white pepper for use at home is quite a safe situation, the use of white pepper when eating out is fraught with problems. It is common practice in the catering trades to use white (wheat) flour in pepperpots to 'make it go further'. One can understand the economy – pepper is an expensive commodity that has to be provided in cafés, restaurants, etc., and mixing it with wheat flour can halve the price. Much safer is the use of black peppercorns and a grinder.

Salt

All types of salt are gluten-free so you have nothing to worry about here.

Cornflour

The word 'cornflour' can cover a multitude of sins. It can be a variety of gluten-free and gluten-containing starches blended together. How are you to know? Find out a brand that is gluten-free and available locally to you. Sometimes 'cornflour' is called 'maize flour'.

Gravy Mixes, Gravy Brownings

These seem particularly susceptible to changes of formula. Look on the label before you buy or, better still, stop using them and go over to using gluten/ wheat-free soy sauces with a thickener such as maize flour. Health stores usually stock a suitable brand.

Q. Are there other things apart from foods that can contain gluten/wheat?

A. Stamps, etc.

Starch, which may contain gluten/wheat, is used in the production of glue for postage stamps and charity stamps, labels, and tapes. I have heard of people who were even allergic to licking these! (The same goes for envelope flaps.)

Sweets

Most types of sweets are gluten- and wheat-free but gluten/wheat-containing flour is used in some to cut down manufacturing costs. Cheap chocolate is suspect; some toffees and chocolate bars with dubious fillings such as little pieces of crunchy biscuit, cream centres and breakfast cereals are all likely to contain gluten or wheat.

Vitamins

If you want to take extra vitamins you must take vitamin tablets or powders which don't use fillers containing gluten or wheat.

Medicines

These too can be made with gluten/wheat-containing starch, especially cough syrups and some drugs in tablet form. Check with your chemist or doctor. If they cannot advise you, write to the manufacturer.

Smoking

There is no gluten in tobacco; however, smoking is a most unhealthy habit. The fact that it is gluten-free is no recommendation to its being a suitable activity for people on a gluten-free diet!

Drinking

A great variety of alcoholic drinks are derived from gluten-containing grains, such as whisky, beers, ales, stouts, barley wine, etc. The not-so-sensitive gluten-free dieter might well be able to drink beer and ale. However, the really safe drinks are those made from fruit and not grains. These are brandies, wines made from grapes, sherry and port.

GLUTEN-FREE SYMBOL

Please note that the use of the universally accepted gluten-free symbol of the crossed grain does not indicate that a product is also wheat-free. It may contain both wheat and starch and a little gluten as this is permitted by law. Such products are not advisable for patients who are allergic to wheat or acutely allergic to gluten.

Gluten-free Symbol

CHAPTER THREE

Gluten-free and Wheat-free Foods to Help You

For those people who are able to eat it, wheat is an extremely good food. It can be grown and harvested all around the world. It has a good taste, is versatile and, more important, it is a nourishing food when used as part of a mixed diet. Small wonder then that it is so widely used in the manufacture of foods and generally in the average diet. Rye, barley and oats are also widely used for the same reasons as wheat.

Fortunately, there are other cereals available, even though they are not as widely used as the four already mentioned.

CEREALS

Sago

Slightly greyish in colour, tastes fairly bland and can be used for milk puddings.

Rice Flour

The most nutritious is made from brown rice but white rice is available too. The coarse version of the flour is called ground rice and can be bought at most grocers and supermarkets. It has only a slight binding ability, but is useful for cookies, crumble topping, pastry and in flour blends. The best binders to use with this are grated apple or dried pectin.

Yellow Split Pea Flour

This is bright yellow in colour and has a very strong pea taste. It contains some pectin and is a better flour for binding than rice. However, its taste is overpowering unless used in small quantities in a flour blend. It is useful for colouring in baking and also in binding. Use ground rice as a substitute if pea flour is difficult to obtain.

Maize Flour

This is made from corn-on-the-cob. It has a creamy colour and can be very finely ground. It has a completely bland taste as it is mainly carbohydrate (not very nutritious). It is also called 'cornflour'. Health shops sell coarsely ground maize flour. This is yellow and called maize meal. It has more taste than the finer flour but is a little too coarse for baking, unless used in small quantities.

Soya Flour

This is a fine, yellow flour, prized for its protein, vitamin E and lecithin content. It has a slightly musty smell and taste and is best used in blends. This should be stored wrapped in the fridge. It binds only slightly but is highly nutritious.

Potato Flour

This is sometimes called 'Farina' and is a fine white starch. It has a slight potato taste, does not bind well and is mainly carbohydrate. However, it combines well with other naturally gluten-free flours.

Trufree Flours

These are made from naturally gluten-free flours and are all wheat-free. Except for the methods of bread making which are much quicker and easier than for wheat bread, the flours handle and bake up like ordinary wheat flour. They all contain binders.

BINDERS

Methylcellulose

Virtually pure fibre, this can be used effectively as a binder in small quantities. It is a dry powder, has a pale creamy grey colour and rather a gritty texture until reconstituted. It has quite a bland taste and is not expensive, but is difficult to obtain.

Dried Pectin

This is expensive but effective and only a small amount is needed. It has a slightly metallic taste to some people.

Grated Apple

This contains pectin and binds particularly well, albeit with an apple taste and a pale green colour. It is a very wet binder and can be used for cakes, pastry, cookies, biscuits, etc. It should be finely grated and include any juice when you weigh it. Grate apples with the peel on as most of the pectin is just under the surface of the peel.

Eggs

These are very useful binders. The white is the part that

actually does the binding, so the yolk can be removed and just the white used effectively if you wish. The trouble with using eggs for binding is that a gluten-free dieter's weekly consumption of eggs could easily be in the region of a dozen, which is really too many. (Eggs are very low in fibre and are frequently blamed for constipation.)

BRANS

Soya Bran

This is best toasted. It is not easy to add to baking and has a very musty taste. However, it is cheap and effective for some in the treatment of constipation. Its colour is yellowy-brown.

Rice Bran

This is made from rice husks and has a quite pleasant bran-type taste. It is useful for adding to biscuits, crumble toppings and bread to increase the fibre content. It does take up a lot of moisture during baking and should only be used in small quantities or it makes the baking taste dry. Some people eat it sprinkled on gluten-free cereal.

'TRUFREE' FLOURS

These are numbered to avoid confusion.

No. 1 for bread which is not only gluten-free and wheat-free but grain-free too.

No. 2 for coarse brown bread with added bran (made from rice husks).

No. 3 for brownbread which has added vitamins and minerals.

No. 4 for white bread, crusty rolls, pizza bases, pasta.

No. 5 for brown bread.

No. 6 a plain flour for pastries and biscuits.

No. 7 a self-raising flour for buns, cakes, biscuits, etc.

This range of flours has been specially designed for people acutely allergic to gluten and/or wheat. They are made in conditions where no contamination can occur from other substances which contain wheat and/or gluten. They are obtainable from chemists and are labelled 'Special Dietary Flour'. A perfectly sound diet can be followed without using these types of flours. i.e. they are not a necessary part of a gluten-free and wheat-free diet. However, they can make such a diet much more varied and interesting and are helpful if a craving for wheat-type products exists as they represent substitutes for wheat flour. (These flours are also lactose-free for coeliacs who also have to follow a lactose-free diet.)

You will find all sorts of recipe methods in this cookbook.

Some will seem peculiar to you, such as making fruit cake with yeast instead of eggs. However, the end results are all palatable and resemble ordinary cooking in appearance, taste, texture, colour, nutrition, so don't be afraid to try recipes, however bizarre they may seem.

A CAUTIONARY NOTE

All the recipes in this book are 100 per cent gluten- and wheat-free and so are suitable for all types of people with a gluten/wheat sensitivity. **Very allergic patients should buy ingredients which have been milled and packed in 'safe' factories where there is no risk of gluten contamination. Remember that manufact- urers can change their formulas at the drop of a hat so please** *check all labels.* By law, in the UK all food products must declare contents on the outside of the pack. Look for a 'box' which gives you these. For example:

Maize, starch, sugar, colouring.

Any of the following can mean the presence of gluten or wheat so be on the look-out for them:

Wholewheat or wholegrain   Rye and rye flour
Wheat and wheat flour   Barley and barley flour
Wheatmeal   Barley flakes
Wheat starch   Barley meal and pearl
Wheat protein   barley

Oat bran
Oats and oat flour
Oat flakes
Oatmeal, pinhead oatmeal
Rolled oats, porridge oats
Edible starch
Special edible starch
Modified starch
Food starch
Special gluten-free food
  starch (usually contains
  wheat starch)
Rusk
Wheat germ
Wheat bran or bran
Durum wheat

Wheat flakes
Kibbled wheat
Flour
Starch
Thickening
Cornflour
Corn
Cornstarch
Binder
Rye flakes
Ryemeal
Cereal
Cereal protein
Vegetable protein
Semolina

Baking

Do not bake ordinary and gluten-free recipes at the same time as it is so easy to make a mistake. Keep gluten-free ingredients separate from ordinary ones to avoid a muddle. (Acutely allergic patients should keep special baking utensils, wooden spoons etc., just for their own baking.)

CHAPTER FOUR

General List of Basic Gluten-free and Wheat-free Items

This list gives a basic framework of 'safe' items. Most can be bought at supermarkets, grocers, greengrocers, butchers or fishmongers. The special flours can be obtained from chemists, some health stores or by mail order. You should be able to use all the bottled and tinned foods on this list without having to worry about which names they carry. Where 'pure' is indicated, you should look for this word on the label; for example, some brands of cheap instant coffee may contain a filler such as wheat. These will not be labelled 'pure' as they are blends. Always check the ingredient box before using any brand.

B
Bacon – all kinds
Beans (dried); haricot, red kidney, etc.
Black treacle
Brandy
Butter

C
Cheese: plain unprocessed kinds such as Cheshire, Edam, Stilton, Cheddar, Brie, Camembert
Cherries (*glacé*) – any colour (always rinse well)

Chopped peel
Cider
Cider vinegar
Coffee (pure)
Cream; tinned, fresh
Crisps (unflavoured)

D
Desiccated coconut
Dried fruit; raisins, sultanas,
    currants, dried fruit salad,
    apricots, etc.

E
Eggs (fresh)

F
Fish; plain fresh, all kinds
Fish; tinned in oil (not
    sauce)
Flaked rice
Flours: Trufree Nos 1 to 7
Fruit; fresh, all kinds
Fruit juices (pure)

G
Golden syrup

H
Honey; thick and thin,
    (pure)

Hemicellulose

J
Jam, all kinds

L
Lemon curd
Lentils; dried

M
Margarine (except those
    with wheat-germ oil)
Marmalade
Meat; fresh, plain
Methylcellulose
Milk; fresh, tinned, dried
Molasses

N
Nuts; all kinds, fresh

P
Pectin (dried)
Pepper; pure white
Peppercorns, whole black
Port (wine)

R
Rice; dried, plain, long and
    short grain or ground
Rice bran

34

Rice flour

S

Salt

Sherry; dry, medium and
  sweet

Soya bran

Soya flour

Soy Sauce; special varieties
  available from health
  stores

Spices (pure); cinnamon,
  allspice, cloves, ginger,
  etc.

Split peas

Sugar; brown and white,
  caster, granulated, icing,

soft brown, moist,
  demerara, fructose, etc.

T

Tapioca

Tea; dried leaves

V

Vegetables; all kinds, fresh

W

Wine; red, white, rosé

Wine vinegar

Y

Yeast extract, Marmite

Yellow split pea flour

BASIC GLUTEN- AND WHEAT-FREE FOODS (ALL FRESH, PLAIN)

- Meat
- Fish
- Eggs
- Fruit

- Vegetables
- Cheese
- Milk
- Rice

CHAPTER FIVE

General List of Gluten- and Wheat-containing Items

Here is a list of ordinary items that you must take care in choosing. They *almost certainly will* contain gluten or wheat although some makes will not – always check the labels for ingredients in the following. See also the list in chapter 3, pages 31–2.

B
Baby foods
Baked beans
Baking powders
Batter mixes
Bedtime drinks
Blancmange
Biscuits and biscuit mixes
Breadcrumbs
Breads
Breakfast cereals
Buns and bun mixes

C
Cakes and cake mixes
Cereals
Chocolate – cheap
 varieties
Chutney
Cocoa
Coffee – instant
Communion wafers
Cornflour
Crispbreads
Crumble topping mix

Curry powder

Custard powder (or tinned custard)

D

Desserts

Drinking chocolate

F

Fish in coating or batter

G

Gravy powder and mixes

I

Ice cream

Instant puddings

M

Macaroni

Malt vinegar (malt may have adverse effects on some dieters)

Mayonnaise

Monosodium glutamate (MSG)

Muesli

Mustard (dry or made up)

O

Oats and oatmeal

P

Pastry mixes

Pasta – vermicelli, lasagne, alphabet spaghetti, tagliatelli, long spaghetti etc.

Paste

Pickles

Pie fillings

Porridge

S

Salad dressings

Sandwich spreads

Sauces

Sausages

Snacks

Soups – tinned and packet mixes

Soy sauce

Spaghetti

Spreads

Stuffing

Suet

Y

Yogurt (fruit flavours)

You will find, by law, a box or special area set aside on each pack for a list of ingredients. Look at this carefully. The ingredients will be in a descending order of amount; e.g. the largest amount of any ingredient first, the smallest last.

It is a good idea to keep a small notebook with names of branded items that you know are gluten-free and easily obtainable in your area. Even so, before you buy, check the ingredients box. Manufacturers can change their formulas without warning.

PROCESSED FOOD

Here is a list of ordinary items which, although gluten-free in their fresh, plain state, can end up containing gluten after processing. (This also applies to wheat.)

Meat

Processed into
    meat pastes or spreads
    sausages
    pâté
    stock cubes
    ham with breadcrumb coating
    beefburgers, rissoles and croquettes
    meat with stuffing (such as oven-ready chicken)
    meat pie fillings
    meat pies and pasties

Fish

Processed into
  fish pastes and spreads
  fish cakes
  fish fingers
  fish in batter
  fish in breadcrumbs } fresh or frozen

Eggs

Processed into
  scotch eggs
  custard tarts
  quiches, flans, pies with egg
  veal and ham pie

Cheese

Processed into
  processed cheese
  sliced cheese
  cheese spreads
  cheese triangles (usually in round flat boxes)
  cheesecake
  cheese snacks (flavoured)

Coffee

Processed into
  cheap instant coffee
  coffee substitutes

Fruit

Processed into
  pie fillings
  fruit yogurt
  desserts
  cheesecake
  sweet sauces

Chocolate

Processed into
  chocolates with centres
  filled bars
  spreads

Nuts

Processed into
  spreads
  coated sweets
  snacks and bars

Milk and Cream

Processed into
   custard (ready-made)
   flavoured drinks
   instant puddings
   ice cream
   yogurt (some flavours)

Spices

Processed into
   cheap spices } these can be mixed with
   curry powder } 'fillers' containing gluten

Tea

Processed into
   instant drinks

Vegetables

Processed into
   frozen vegetables such as chips
   sauces (savoury)
   pickles, chutney

Oils

Processed into
  salad dressings, mayonnaise

CHAPTER SIX

Emergency Gluten-free
and Wheat-free Menus

Rarely, if ever, does a gluten-free and/or wheat-free diet come with fair warning. It is more likely to be thrust suddenly into one's life, bringing with it all the confusion and upheaval one would expect. It is not an easy task to gain a full understanding of the problem and adjust immediately. There will be a gap of perhaps two or three days in which sources of supply for new and strange ingredients have to be tracked down. Without the broad knowledge that experience brings, mistakes are likely, especially in the first few weeks of going on to a new type of diet.

The following suggestions for an eating pattern may help someone thrown in at the deep end who will not have had time to buy special items needed. They are also a useful guide to eating out where specialized food is unobtainable. Eat only the food suggested and these menus are quite safe to use.

BASIC MENU FOR BEGINNERS

Breakfast

Fried potatoes; grilled bacon and fried or poached egg; pure fruit juice such as orange, grapefruit; tea and coffee with milk. *Do not be tempted to eat bread or breakfast cereals unless you know they are gluten/wheat-free.*

Lunch

Boiled potatoes or potatoes baked in their jackets; salad of tomatoes, lettuce, cucumber, grated carrot; tinned salmon or tuna or sardines – all fish must be canned in *oil* and not in some kind of sauce. Use a dressing, if required, of thin cooking oil, lemon juice, a little sugar, salt and black pepper. For a sweet, eat any kind of fresh fruit such as apples, pears, bananas.

Dinner

Grilled chop, either lamb or pork; plain boiled greens of some kind; plain rice, boiled. Make gravy with the juices of the meat with its fat drained off and water strained from the vegetables. *Do not use any kind of gravy mix.* For sweet eat more fruit.

Snacks

Do not eat any bought cakes, biscuits, pastries. Allow yourself up to three bananas per day.

Obviously, this represents a very narrow outlook on the diet and is only for use in an emergency. At least all the food is perfectly safe. You may find that you will have to eat more rice and potatoes than you would normally, so increase the portions of these. You will have no worries about ingredients of foods if you stick to plain fresh foods at this stage of the proceedings.

Eating out is always a problem and should be avoided in the early days of going on to the diet. Even the most experienced exclusion dieter can get caught out by unusual foods.

SUGGESTED MENUS INCLUDING SPECIAL FOODS (LONG-TERM DIET)

Breakfasts

Fruit juice; slice of back bacon grilled with tomatoes; special bread toasted, suitable margarine and marmalade; tea or coffee with milk.

½ grapefruit with sugar; egg (boiled, scrambled, poached or baked); special bread, toasted or fried and suitable margarine; tea or coffee with milk.

Special muesli with fresh fruit and nuts etc. (see recipe); tea or coffee with milk.

Fruit juice; gluten/wheat-free baked beans on special toast with margarine; gluten/wheat-free cereal with milk and sugar; tea or coffee with milk.

Apple or pear; special toast with suitable margarine; fried mushrooms and grilled back bacon; tea or coffee with milk.

(People who cannot face breakfast should take a milk-based drink such as ½ pint (275ml) milk blended with a banana, 1 to 2 teaspoonsful honey, a few sunflower seeds.)

Lunches

Large mixed salad with oil/vinegar dressing; slice of cold beef, ham (without breadcrumb coating), cold pork, cold chicken or similar; or, cheese, hard boiled eggs, tinned sardines, salmon or tuna fish; potato baked in its jacket with margarine; finish with fresh fruit of some kind.

Bowl of special home-made soup; slice of toasted cheese on special bread; fresh or stewed fruit to follow, or piece of special fruit cake.

Teas (if eaten)

Snack made with special bread such as sandwiches filled with cucumber or tomato slices. Either cake or buns made with special flour (see recipes).

Dinners

Either rice or potatoes (boiled, roast, chipped or baked) and one or two green vegetables, lightly cooked, (kale, cabbage, broccoli, green beans, peas etc.) Also have grilled, roasted or casserole-cooked meat of some kind; or fresh fish (grilled, steamed, fried or casseroled).

GENERAL CONSIDERATIONS

You should eat at least one or two large helpings of 'greens' every day and a mixed salad, plus some fresh fruit. Include at least two portions of high-protein food such as meat or fish. The main starches should be potatoes and rice, topped up with special bread, pastry and cakes. If the last three cannot be afforded then the amount of rice and potatoes should be increased, otherwise there could be a sudden weight loss which may be difficult to regain.

If loss of appetite results in an unbalanced diet, it is a good idea to supplement with extra vitamins and minerals. As the ordinary kind will almost certainly have wheat- or gluten-containing fillers in their composition, special ones will have to be taken. The following products are gluten-free and wheat-free and are designed specially for people on exclusion diets who need to *supplement* their diet:

Trufree vitamins and minerals.

(The most likely occurring deficiency in a diet low in grains will be B-complex vitamins: B_1, B_2, B_3, calcium pantothenate, B_6, inositol, choline, B_{12}, folic acid, PABA and biotin.)

Snacks should only be eaten if there is no danger of becoming overweight. Plain nuts, fresh fruit, carrot sticks, dried fruit and special biscuits and buns can be eaten. Children should be encouraged not to eat junk snack foods such as candy and chocolate bars, crisps, etc.

MENUS FOR CHILDREN

These menus feature readily obtainable foods and require no specialized shopping:

Breakfasts

Grilled bacon, tomatoes, fried (cold boiled) potatoes; fruit juice, tea with milk or milk

Grilled bacon, fried or poached egg, fried mushrooms; fruit juice, tea with milk or milk.

Home-made fish cakes (see recipes), grilled tomatoes; fresh orange segments with sugar; tea with milk or milk.

Snacks

Bananas, apples, pears, oranges.

Lunches

Fresh cod, haddock or plaice, dipped in ground rice and fried in cooking oil; peas, carrots, chipped fresh potatoes fried in cooking oil; Baked Apple (see recipes).

Grilled lamb chop, fresh boiled greens, carrots or swede, boiled potatoes or plain boiled rice; stewed fresh fruit such as apple or Baked Bananas (see recipes).

Chicken casserole for one; fresh fruit salad (see recipes).

Suppers

Salad of lettuce, cucumber, grated carrot, tomato, plus tinned salmon, sardines or tuna fish in *oil* – drain off the oil – (see recipe for Salad Dressing); baked jacket potato with butter or margarine.

Baked beans (Heinz), chipped potatoes, poached egg.

Savoury rice and plain omelette or scrambled egg (see recipes).

(If a *wheat-free* diet only has to be followed, you may include some rye crispbreads, but these are not suitable for *gluten-free* diets.)

These suggestions are suitable for the whole family and so there is no need to cook two separate lots of food. The other members of the family can add ordinary bread etc. to the menus, but care should be taken not to put temptation in the way of a child on a special diet, especially in the early stages of transition to the new diet.

Try to make the child's food colourful and attractive, whilst providing variety and sound nutrition. Green vegetables should be eaten every day. Most children love chipped potatoes, but avoid giving these too often. Limit eggs to one per day. Margarine (provided it contains no wheat-germ oil) or butter can be used with potatoes, or other boiled vegetables. Tea, pure coffee, milk and fruit juices can also be used as snacks throughout the day. Give home-made lemonade (see recipes) instead of bought orange or lemon drinks.

These emergency menus only give a basic framework to the diet, which can be broadened by the addition of special bread, cake, biscuits, puddings and snacks. Also use the long-term menus suggested for adults to broaden the diet.

CHAPTER SEVEN

Recipes

The recipes which follow are all gluten- and wheat-free; they are suitable for coeliacs and wheat sensitive or allergic patients. Recipes marked with a star * are made with ingredients readily available at most grocers, supermarkets, greengrocers etc., i.e. they do not require any specialized ingredients. These recipes may be used to expand the emergency menus as a stepping stone to the very specialized recipes which require sometimes difficult shopping and which nobody would expect to be able to organize immediately.

SAVOURY RECIPES

Special Breadcrumbs

There are two ways to make these from stale special bread. Either finely grate slices of bread or break them up into an electric grinder such as you would use to grind coffee beans. Grind for a few seconds only, or the crumbs will be too fine. Sprinkle on to a baking sheet and dry slowly in the oven for a couple of hours on a very low heat. Allow to cool and store in an air-tight jar in the fridge. Use, as required, for coating fish cakes and fish after dipping in beaten egg. There is no need to dry out the crumbs if they are to be used immediately.

*Fish Cakes (makes 6)

    8 oz (225g) cod, haddock or coley, boned and washed
    Juice of ½ lemon
    8 oz (225g) cold boiled potato
    1 oz (25g) margarine
    1 tablespoonful freshly chopped parsley
    Salt and pepper
    Oil for frying

Put the fish into a saucepan and pour over a little water. Cook with the lid on for 6-8 minutes. Strain off the excess liquid. In a mixing bowl, mash the potato with the margarine. Add all the other ingredients and mix with a fork until the fish is evenly distributed. With the hands, form flat round cakes. Fry in hot shallow oil for 3 minutes on each side.

*Mashed Potato

Cook potatoes in boiling salted water for about 25 minutes, or until soft enough to mash. Strain and return to the saucepan. Mash well, taking care to eliminate any lumps. Add 1 teaspoonful of butter or suitable margarine per portion and a dash of milk. Beat to a cream with a wooden spoon. Season to taste and add 1 or 2 pinches of ground nutmeg. Beat again and serve hot.

With the exclusion of wheat, the diet relies more heavily on potatoes and rice as a source of carbohydrate than an ordinary diet. It is very important to make the most of potatoes, otherwise they can be a very boring and tasteless vegetable. Rice can be made much more exciting by adding a variety of cooked diced vegetables. These will vary according to the season.

*Savoury Rice

>   1 medium onion, peeled and chopped
>   1½ oz (40g) margarine
>   ½ green pepper, de-seeded and chopped
>   1 medium carrot, scrubbed and diced
>   1 stick celery, scrubbed and chopped
>   3 sprigs watercress *or* 3 spinach leaves, stalks
>   removed and torn into small pieces
>   1 cup cooked rice (1 portion)
>   Salt and pepper to taste

Fry the onion gently in the margarine. Add the prepared vegetables and a little water to prevent sticking. Cook with the lid on for 8-10 minutes. Add the cooked rice and heat through, mixing everything together with a wooden spoon. Serve hot.

The vegetables can be varied according to season and taste.

Yorkshire Pudding

Makes 12 small or 1 large and is suitable for all the family.

    4 oz (100g) Trufree No. 7 Flour
    3 pinches of salt
    1 egg
    1 tablespoonful cooking oil
    ½ pint (275ml) milk
    Oil for baking tins

Preheat the oven to 475°F/240°C (Gas Mark 9). Put the flour, salt and tablespoonful of oil into a bowl. Mix and make a well in the centre. Break the egg into it and stir into the flour. Gradually add the milk and stir in, beating as soon as you are able, to form a milky batter. Heat 2 to 3 tablespoonsful oil in a baking tin or patty tins. Pour in the batter, using a spoon for the small ones. Bake for 5 minutes and then lower the heat to 425°F/220°C (Gas Mark 7). Continue baking for another 30 minutes and serve immediately with roast beef.

Gravy

Strain the fat off meat juices from the grill or roasting tin. Sprinkle in about 2 heaped teaspoonsful gluten-free cornflour or maize flour. Rub in with a wooden spoon and, while cooking, gradually add the strainings from the vegetables (if any) or water. Add 2 teaspoonsful gluten/wheat-free soy sauce and bring to the boil. Simmer while stirring for 2 minutes and the gravy is ready to serve.

It is nonsense to suppose that good gravy can only be made with a gravy mix or stock cube. The very best gravy is always made with the meat juices (not the fat) and thickened slightly with some kind of flour, then thinned down with vegetable stocks.

Emergency Thickening or Stock for Gravy

Take half a boiled potato and mash thoroughly with a fork. Add this to meat juices with the fat strained off, with ¼ teaspoonful of Marmite (optional) and some water strained from boiled vegetables. Stir well with a wooden spoon and bring back to the boil. Simmer for a minute while stirring and season to taste. Serve hot.

If you have any stock available, such as the brown juice that forms underneath cold dripping from a roast joint, add this instead of the Marmite.

*Salad Dressing

½ level teaspoonful salt
Good dash freshly ground black pepper
2 tablespoonsful wine or cider vinegar
3 tablespoonsful oil – sunflower, soya or corn are
   suitable
1 level tablespoonful soft brown sugar

Put all the ingredients into a screw-top jar and shake well
to combine. Store it in the fridge and shake well again
before using.

Chicken Casserole for One

This is an easy main meal for one person and useful if the
rest of the family is to eat something quite different.

½ medium onion
2 teaspoonsful cooking oil
1 mushroom
1 carrot
1 small tin tomatoes
Gluten/wheat-free soy sauce
1 boned chicken breast
1 large potato
Couple of chopped parsley sprigs or a pinch of drired
   rosemary

Preheat the oven to 400°F/200°C (Gas Mark 6). Fry the sliced onion in the oil until transparent. Add the sliced mushroom, carrot and tomatoes and bring to the boil. Mix in 2 teaspoonsful of soy sauce and transfer to a warmed casserole. Stir and lay the chicken breast in the centre. Cover with layers of thickly sliced potato. Season with salt and freshly ground black pepper. Sprinkle with the chosen herb and put the lid on. Bake for about an hour. Spoon onto a warm plate and serve.

Home-made Vegetable Soup

A hearty family soup.

> 2 teaspoonsful cooking oil
> ½ medium onion, peeled and sliced
> 1 medium carrot, scrubbed and sliced thickly
> ½ stick of celery, washed and cut into pieces
> ½ medium turnip, peeled and cut into pieces
> ½ medium potato, peeled and sliced thickly
> 4 sprouts, prepared and sliced in half
> ¾ pint (425ml) water
> 2 teaspoonsful gluten/wheat-free soy sauce
> Salt and black pepper to taste

Fry the onion gently in the oil for 3 to 4 minutes in a saucepan with the lid on. Add all the other vegetables and half of the water plus the soy sauce. Bring to the boil and simmer for 15 minutes to soften the vegetables. Add the remaining water and pour into the liquidizer goblet.

Blend and return to the pan. Heat through, season to taste and simmer for 2 minutes. Serve hot. If it tastes slightly bitter then add about ½ teaspoonful of sugar. Dilute if it turns out too thick, using more water.

Water Biscuits

    4 oz (100g) Trufree No. 6 plain flour
    1 oz (25g) soft margarine
    2 pinches salt
    Cold water
    Extra flour for rolling out (Trufree No. 6 as above or
        maize flour

Preheat the oven to 450°F/230°C (Gas Mark 8). Put the flour and salt into a basin with the margarine and rub in until the mixture resembles breadcrumbs. Add about 1 tablespoonful of cold water and mix with a fork to a stiff paste, adding more water if required. Knead quickly, using more of the flour, into one lump of soft dough. Roll out, using more of the flour, and cut into squares. Place on baking sheets with a spatula. Prick with a fork and bake for about 8 to 10 minutes on the top shelf of the oven until golden. (Do not overbake, they should be pale in colour.) Makes about 15 biscuits. Cool on a wire rack and store in a tin when cold.

*Savoury Straws

1 oz (25g) cold mashed potatoes
½ oz (15g) soft margarine
Pinch of salt
2 oz (50g) ground rice
1 level teaspoonful very finely chopped onion

Preheat the oven to 425°F/220°C (Gas Mark 7). Put the potato and margarine into a bowl and beat to a cream. Gradually add the salt, ground rice and onion and combine with a fork. Knead by hand into one ball, adding a little ground rice, and cut into fingers after rolling out. Place on an ungreased baking sheet and bake until golden – about 10 minutes. Cool on a baking sheet. Eat on the day of baking. These taste particularly good with soup.

BREADS

Brown Bread

10½ oz (290g) Trufree No. 5 flour
¼ oz (7g) instant yeast
3 teaspoonsful cooking oil
8 fl oz (225ml) warm water

Preheat the oven to 350°F/180°C (Gas Mark 4). Put the flour into a bowl and sprinkle in the yeast. Stir well and add the cooking oil and the warm water. Stir to a thick batter with a wooden spoon. Grease a loaf tin (7¼ × 3½ × 2¼ in. or 185 × 90 × 50mm). Pour the batter into the prepared tin immediately and place in the oven on the top shelf. Bake for approximately one hour when the loaf should be well-risen, golden brown and crusty. As soon as it is baked, turn it out of the tin and cool on a wire rack. Cut when cold and use as ordinary bread.

This bread is made in a completely different way to ordinary wheat bread. There is no kneading or proving to do and so it is very quick to make. Use as ordinary bread – fry, toast, make into breadcrumbs etc. (This recipe may also be used with Trufree No. 5 flour for White Bread.)

White Bread

> 9 fl oz (250ml) warm water
> 2 slightly heaped teaspoonsful dried yeast granules
> 1 heaped teaspoonful sugar
> 1 oz (25g) soya flour
> 4½ oz (115g) potato flour
> ¾ oz (20g) yellow split pea flour
> ¾ oz (20g) ground almonds or hazelnuts
> 2 level teaspoonsful dried pectin (to bind)
> 3 pinches of salt
> 3 tablespoons cooking oil

Preheat the oven to 350°F/180°C (Gas Mark 4). Sprinkle the yeast into the warm water with the sugar and leave to soften for a few minutes. Put all other ingredients into a bowl and mix well with the hands, breaking up any lumps. Stir the yeast, water and sugar and pour onto the flour mixture. Mix, then beat with a wooden spoon. (Do not use an electric beater as this will make the loaf tough.) Grease a medium-sized loaf tin with oil and flour with potato or maize flour. Pour the mixture into this and put straight into the oven on the top shelf. After baking for one hour it should be well risen, golden and crusty. Turn out onto a wire rack to cool and do not cut until cold.

Use as ordinary bread, but keep it stored in a clean plastic bag away from other bread. This should give about 3 days' supply. (The tin size should be the same as for the Brown Bread recipe.)

SWEET RECIPES

Pastry Tartlets

4 oz (100g) Trufree No. 6 plain flour
1½ oz (40g) soft margarine
2 tablespoonsful cold water
extra No. 6 flour for rolling out etc.

Preheat the oven to 425°F/220°C (Gas Mark 7). Put the flour and margarine into a bowl and blend with a fork to start with. Then rub in with the fingers until the mixture resembles breadcrumbs. Add the 2 tablespoonsful of cold water and mix until it forms one large lump. Sprinkle in more flour and finish kneading it by hand. Roll out, using more flour. Cut into rounds and use a spatula to place into patty tins – the half-round type are easiest to use. Bake for about 10 minutes on the top shelf. Fill with jam or sweetened stewed fruit when cold.

*Baked Bananas (Serves 4)

4 bananas, peeled and cut in half lengthways
3 oz (75g) soft brown sugar
Juice of 2 small oranges
1 oz (25g) butter or margarine

Put the halved bananas in a warmed ovenproof dish. Sprinkle with the sugar and pour over the orange juice. Dot with the butter or margarine. Bake in a preheated oven at 350°F/180°C (Gas Mark 4) for about 15 minutes. Serve hot. For a treat, top with a little single cream.

*Baked Apple

1 large cooking apple
Water
A few sultanas
1–2 heaped teaspoonsful soft brown sugar

Wash the apple and cut out the core, leaving the apple whole. Cut a line round the middle as the flesh will expand during baking. Place in an ovenproof dish and pour over about ¾ cupful of water. Put the sultanas into the hole left by removing the core and sprinkle with the sugar. Bake at 350°F/180°C (Gas Mark 4) on the middle shelf for about half an hour. Serve hot.

*Fruit Tart

For the pastry:
> 2 oz (50g) soft margarine
> 4 oz (100g) ground rice
> 3 oz (75g) finely grated eating apple

For the filling:
> 5 or 6 oz (150–175g) stewed fruit, sweetened with brown sugar – if the fruit is too liquid then thicken with maize flour.

Use a fork to blend the three pastry ingredients. Knead by hand until they form one ball in the bowl. Grease an enamel or glass ovenproof plate and put the dough in the centre. Flatten with the palm of the hand and fingers until it has spread evenly all over the bottom. Raise a slight edge all round, pinching with the thumb and forefinger. Spread with the fruit mixture and bake in a preheated oven at 425°F/220°C (Gas Mark 7) for 20 to 25 minutes, near the top of the oven. Cut into slices and eat hot or cold. The pastry will crispen up as the tart cools down.

*Fruit Cookies

2 oz (50g) soft margarine
4 oz (100g) ground rice
3 oz (75g) finely grated eating apple
1½ oz (40g) brown sugar
1½ oz (40g) dried fruit
½ teaspoonful mixed spice (gluten-free and wheat-free)

Preheat the oven to 450°F/230°C (Gas Mark 8). Blend the margarine and ground rice with a fork. Add the apple *mush*, sugar, spice and dried fruit. Knead and mix with a wooden spoon until one large ball of dough has formed. Grease a baking sheet with margarine and drop spoons of the dough on to it. Spread out with a knife into biscuit shapes about ¼ in. thick. Bake above the centre of the oven for about 20 to 25 minutes. Allow to cool for a minute and then remove with a spatula. The cookies will go crisp as they cool down. Eat within two days.

To add variation, omit the spice and substitute 1 heaped teaspoonful of grated orange or lemon rind.

Rich Fruit Cake

(Suitable for birthday cake, Christmas cake etc.)

8 oz (225g) Trufree No. 7 flour
¼ level teaspoonful salt
1 level teaspoonful mixed spice

1 level teaspoon cinnamon
2 oz (50g) ground almonds
4 oz (100g) brown sugar
6 oz (175g) soft margarine
2 generous teaspoonsful black treacle
3 eggs
2 tablespoonsful sherry
1 lb (450g) dried mixed fruit
2 oz (50g) raisins
2 oz (50g) glacé cherries
Grated rind of 1 lemon

Preheat the oven to 325°F/170°C (Gas Mark 3). Mix the flour, salt and spices with the ground almonds. In a large bowl cream the sugar, margarine and treacle. Beat the eggs and sherry in a small bowl and add alternately with the flour mixture to the margarine mixture. When all the mixtures are combined, stir in all the fruit and rind. Line a 7 in. cake tin with greased greaseproof paper. Put the cake mixture into this and flatten it with a knife. Bake on the middle shelf for 1¼ hours. After this, lower the heat to 300°F/150°C (Gas Mark 2) and cook until baked. Cool in the tin for several hours. Turn out carefully and store in a large air-tight tin until required. When needed, remove the greaseproof paper. Spread the cake with apricot jam, cover with gluten- and wheat-free marzipan and ice with royal icing. Serve on a cake board decorated appropriately.

It is doubtful whether anyone could tell the difference between this cake and one made with wheat flour, so do not be afraid to hand it round to the rest of the family and save having to make two types of cakes. If you prefer a very moist cake, prick the top of the cake with a fork and dribble in more sherry. Do this three days running before you ice it.

Pancakes (makes 3)

2 oz (50g) Trufree No. 7 flour
1 egg
¼ pint (140ml) milk
Pinch of salt
1 teaspoonful caster sugar
Oil for frying

Put the flour and egg into a basin and mix to a stiff paste. Gradually add the milk, making sure you get all the lumps out. Beat in the salt and sugar. Heat the frying pan and pour in a little oil. Pour in one third of the batter, tilting the pan to cover all the base. Cook until it will shift if shaken. Either toss or turn over with a spatula to cook the other side. Serve immediately with lemon and sugar, or, spread with jam, rolled up.

Rock Buns

5 oz (140g) Trufree No. 7 flour
2½ oz (70h) soft margarine
2½ oz (70g) brown sugar
1 egg beaten

4 oz (100g) dried mixed fruit
Grated rind of 1 lemon or orange

Preheat the oven to 425°F/220°C (Gas Mark 7). Put the flour and margarine into a bowl and rub in until they resemble fine breadcrumbs. Stir in the sugar and then the egg. Mix to a sticky paste. Add the fruit and rind and mix again. Grease a baking sheet with margarine and Trufree flour, maize or potato flour. Put spoonfuls of the mixture onto the tray, leaving space for the buns to spread. Sprinkle with a little more sugar and bake on the top shelf for 12 to 15 minutes. Do not bake them brown – they should be light golden in colour. Cool on a wire rack and eat freshly baked, preferably while still warm. Use at tea-time or as a snack.

Sponge Buns (makes 6 buns)

2 oz (50g) brown sugar
2 oz (50g) soft margarine
1 egg
2½ oz (65g) Trufree No. 7 flour

Preheat the oven to 375°F/190°C (Gas Mark 5). Put 6 small cake papers into 6 patty tins, or grease and flour the patty tins. Place all the ingredients in a bowl and mix to a soft, creamy consistency. Spoon into the cake papers or patty tins and bake on the top shelf for 15 to 18 minutes. Remove the cakes from the tins and cool on a wire rack. Use at tea-time or for snacks.

These are easy and quick to make. They can be flavoured in all kinds of ways. Add any *one* of the following: 1 heaped teaspoonful grated orange or lemon rind; ½ level teaspoonful dried ginger; 1 tablespoonful currants or sultanas or mixed fruit; 1 heaped teaspoonful gluten-free and wheat-free instant coffee, 1 heaped teaspoonful gluten-free and wheat-free cocoa.

Dundee Cake

¼ pint (140ml) unsweetened orange juice
1 heaped tablespoonful brown sugar
¼ oz (7g) dried yeast
3 tablespoonsful cooking oil (scant)
3 oz (75g) eating apple – wash but do not peel or core
1½ oz (40g) fresh carrot scrubbed and sliced

Flour blend:
1 oz (25g) soya flour
5 oz (115g) ground rice
1 teaspoonful mixed spice (gluten- and wheat-free)
2 oz (50g) ground almonds

Fruit:
8 oz (225g) dried fruit
Grated rind of 1 lemon and 1 orange

Decoration:
1 oz (25g) split almonds

Preheat the oven to 350°F/180°C (Gas Mark 4). In a small saucepan, warm the fruit juice very gently. When it becomes lukewarm, pour into the liquidizer goblet and sprinkle in the dried yeast and leave to soften for a few minutes. Make the flour up in a mixing bowl and stir in the sugar and oil. Add the apple and carrot pieces to the yeast/juice in the liquidizer. Blend and pour over the flour mix. Stir well and then put in all the fruit and rinds. Mix really well until the fruit is evenly distributed. Grease either a Pyrex *soufflé* dish or a cake tin about 7 in diameter (17.5cm) with margarine. Spoon in the cake mixture and flatten the top with a knife. Decorate neatly with the split almonds pressing them slightly into the surface. Bake for about 1 hour at the top of the oven. Test with a knife or a skewer to see if the cake is done. If it needs longer, cover with greaseproof paper and put back in the oven with the heat on a lower setting for a few more minutes. Leave in the dish or tin to cool.

This is a lovely moist cake which keeps for up to two weeks. It is very difficult to distinguish from one made in the traditional way with wheat flour and eggs.

Shortbread Biscuits

    3 oz (75g) butter
    2 oz (50g) caster sugar
    ½ beaten egg
    7 oz (200g) Trufree No. 6 flour
    2 pinches of salt
    Cold water
    Extra Trufree No. 6 flour for rolling out etc.

Preheat the oven to 350°F/180°C (Gas Mark 4). Cream the butter and sugar. Add the egg and mix well. Sprinkle in the flour and salt and mix to a stiff paste using a wooden spoon. Add a little cold water if needed. Use more flour to knead into one ball of dough. Roll out to just over ⅛ inch thick (4mm) and cut into about 30 biscuits. Place on baking sheets and prick with a fork or skewer. Bake until golden (not browning) for about 20 minutes in the middle of the oven. Cool on a wire rack and, when cold, store in an air-tight container.

Muesli

The traditional version of this type of breakfast has a base of oats and cannot be used. However, by changing the base, a delicious breakfast can be enjoyed.

Assemble all the ingredients in a bowl and pour on cold milk or, if preferred, fruit juice. For a base use cold cooked rice – about 1 heaped tablespoonful. Sprinkle into a cereal bowl. Slice a banana into it, half an apple (eating variety), a few raisins, almonds or hazelnuts, sunflower and sesame seeds. According to season, other kinds of fresh fruit can be added such as a few raspberries or strawberries. Dried fruits such as apricots can be used if chopped small. Some people prefer a non-sweet kind of breakfast but those who need something sweeter will like to top the muesli with either a little runny honey or a spinkle of brown sugar.

*Fruit Crumble

> 1 portion stewed fruit, sweetened with brown sugar
>   to taste
> 1½ oz (40g) soft margarine
> ½ oz (15g) ground almonds
> 2 oz (50g) ground rice
> ½ oz (15g) brown sugar

Preheat the oven to 425°F/220°C (Gas Mark 7). Put the stewed fruit into a small ovenproof dish and flatten the top evenly. Put all other ingredients into a mixing bowl and rub in the margarine until the mixture resembles breadcrumbs. Spoon gently on to the stewed fruit, covering it all over. Make a hole through to the fruit in the centre, to let out the steam during cooking. Bake near the top of the oven for ten minutes until just browning. Serve hot or cold.

Choose stewing fruit from either fresh or dried varieties – dried apricots, prunes, mixed fruit salad or fresh fruits in season such as apricots, plums, gooseberries, blackcurrants, blackberry and apple, stewing pears, cooking apples, rhubarb etc.

DRINKS

*Lemonade

Thoroughly wash 2 lemons. Cut into slices, including the peel and place in a large jug. Pour about 1 pint (550ml) boiling water over the slices, and sprinkle in 1 tablespoonful of soft brown sugar. Leave to stand for about 12 hours or overnight. Strain and use the resulting juice, diluted with water to taste.

This method can be used with oranges but the flavour will not be so strong. Oranges and lemons can also make a refreshing combination.

*Milk Shakes

½ pint (275ml) milk
1 banana (or other fruit)
1 teaspoonful brown sugar

Place all the ingredients in a liquidizer and blend. Pour into a tall glass and serve immediately.

Other fresh fruits can be used singly or in combinations; strawberries, raspberries, grapes (with pips removed), fresh pineapple (1 slice), cherries (with stones removed), eating apples, pears, plums (stones removed), peaches and nectarines (stones removed). Stewed fruit may also be used. The best ratio is about 2 tablespoonsful of stewed fruit to about ½ pint milk. Add brown sugar to taste.

Useful Information

The following books contain wheat-free and gluten-free recipes:

Beyond the Staff of Life, Kief Adler, Thorsons.
The Bumper Bake Book, the cookbook for *Trufree* flours, Trufree Foods, 225 Putney Bridge Road, London SW15 2PY.
Gluten Free Cooking, Rita Greer, Thorsons.
Wheat Free, Milk Free, Egg Free Cooking, Rita Greer, Thorsons.

Larkhall Natural Health makes a special range of gluten-free and wheat-free flours (also vitamins and minerals) called *Trufree*. Details can be obtained from the Trufree Foods Dept., 225 Putney Bridge Road, London SW15 2PY. All *Trufree* products are made in conditions where no wheat or gluten are present to contaminate them. Other naturally gluten-free and wheat-free foods can be obtained from health food stores and ordinary grocers. Large chemists often stock Trufree flours.

Supplements (*Trufree* vitamins and minerals) available from Health Food Stores, Chemists or by mail order. Ask your medical practitioner or dietitian where you can obtain a list of brands that are gluten/wheat free.

Index

Also available:

Diets to help
ASTHMA AND HAY FEVER
Suitable for all catarrhal conditions

Roger Newman Turner

Asthma and hay fever can be made worse by eating certain foods, but there are also nutritional guidelines that you can follow to help *manage* the condition. This book explains:

- why some people are prone to asthma or hay fever
- how to cut down on mucus-forming foods
- how to increase your intake of protective vitamins and minerals

It includes basic diets to help control the condition and specific diets for more acute symptoms.

ROGER NEWMAN TURNER is a leading naturopath, osteopath and acupuncturist. He has many years' experience treating a wide range of conditions and runs practices in Harley Street, London and Letchworth, Hertfordshire.

Diets to help
CYSTITIS
Total relief without antibiotics

Ralph McCutcheon

Cystitis is an irritating and often chronic infection of the urinary system which does not always respond to symptomatic treatment through antibiotics

This book offers a full nutritional approach to help restore the body's underlying health and avoid cystitis completely. It explains:

- what causes cystitis
- the complementary treatments that can help
- the importance of a balanced diet
- how to cope with an acute attack

It also includes a selection of basic recipes, advice on mineral intake and suggests which foods will help and which foods to avoid.

RALPH McCUTCHEON is a naturopath, osteopath and acupuncturist with many years' experience treating a wide range of conditions with complementary medicine. His practice is near Belfast, Northern Ireland.

DIETS TO HELP ARTHRITIS	0 7225 2871 X	£2.99	☐
DIETS TO HELP ASTHMA AND HAY FEVER	0 7225 2911 2	£2.99	☐
DIETS TO HELP COLITIS	0 7225 3199 0	£2.99	☐
DIETS TO HELP CONTROL CHOLESTEROL	0 7225 2932 5	£2.99	☐
DIETS TO HELP CYSTITIS	0 7225 2872 8	£2.99	☐
DIETS TO HELP DIABETICS	0 7225 2933 3	£2.99	☐
DIETS TO HELP MULTIPLE SCLEROSIS	0 7225 3239 3	£2.99	☐
DIETS TO HELP PSORIASIS	0 7225 2929 5	£2.99	☐

All these books are available from your local bookseller or can be ordered direct from the publishers.

To order direct just tick the titles you want and fill in the form below:

Name: _____

Address:_____

_____

_____ **Postcode:** _____

Send to: Thorsons Mail Order, Dept 3, HarperCollins*Publishers***, Westerhill Road, Bishopbriggs, Glasgow G64 2QT.**
Please enclose a cheque or postal order or your authority to debit your Visa/Access account —

Credit card no: _____

Expiry date: _____

Signature:_____

— up to the value of the cover price plus:
UK & BFPO: Add £1.00 for the first book and 25p for each additional book ordered.
Overseas orders including Eire: Please add £2.95 service charge. Books will be sent by surface mail but quotes for airmail despatches will be given on request.

24 HOUR TELEPHONE ORDERING SERVICE FOR ACCESS/VISA CARDHOLDERS — TEL: 0141 772 2281.